MW00892661

Kicking My AS:

*Life and Lessons
of
Ankylosing Spondylitis*

by Kip Jennings

Copyright © 2013 Kip Jennings

All rights reserved.

ISBN: 1494252988
ISBN-13: 978-1494252984

CONTENTS

To Mary, Robert and Lindsay.
Where would I be without you?

INTRODUCTION

At 8:12 on a sunny, September morning my doctor's assistant called. "How far are you away from a hospital?" she asked. And so began what would ultimately be my life with Ankylosing Spondylitis, also known as AS.

AS literally impacts millions of American lives, yet is a disease very few people have heard of, let alone understand. Mention "cancer" to someone and they inevitably say, "Oh!" Say "Ankylosing Spondylitis" to that same person and they'll say, "Huh?" While the lack of knowledge of AS is understandable, it leads to misunderstandings and, ultimately, frustrations for not only the millions of sufferers AS but their friends, family and acquaintances.

What follows is a brief journey through Ankylosing Spondylitis, or AS. It is intended for both the sufferers of AS and their loved ones, and is an abridged version of what I've experienced, what it is, what sufferers say and – ultimately – how it has made me a better person. It is a story of information, frustration and – ideally – hope.

Please note I am not a physician. I'm not even an expert. You should rely on your doctor more than me. But this is my experience and what I've gleaned over the past year.

This is the first of what will be two versions. Please feel free to send me your questions, comments, insights or corrections at kipejennings@yahoo.com. I would love to incorporate your feedback into the 2nd Edition, and am happy to alert you when the next version is released.

PREFACE: GRANDMA

In the early days, I liked my grandma.

She watched us during summer vacation, bought two presents for each grandchild at Christmas and liked sports. For a young boy, those were good things.

But my parents disliked – if not downright detested -- her.

"Grandma's nice," I said to my mother one day.

"She's *not* nice," my mother retorted. "She was abusive."

For many years, my mom told tales of a childhood spent with a monstrous woman who screamed at her kids, lashed at them with a hair brush and would spend long days laying on the couch.

At some point, the stories had an effect. Suddenly, I started seeing all my grandma's faults. The inactivity. The bitterness. And the endless complaints about aches and pains.

When she walked, she walked painfully slow, hunched over and with bent knees. *I'm old*, she'd say.

It's because she didn't take care of her herself, we'd say. *If she'd get off the couch, she'd feel better*, we told ourselves.

Over time, I disliked her. Then detested her. I barely spoke to her the last 10 years of her life, and when she died in hospice, none of her four children or her countless grandchildren were by her side.

I never felt guilty - it was her own fault.

You make your own bed, I told myself. No matter how tired she was, no matter how much she ached, she could have overcame it if she wanted to. I believed – always – that where there was a will, there was a way.

She simply didn't care enough.

Or so I believed...

PART 1:   MY STORY

A HEALTHY MIDDLE AGED MAN

For my entire adult life, I was healthy.

Actually, *off the charts* healthy. I was 40 and could *easily* do my age in pushups, ran wind sprints every morning and played softball like a 25-year old. I was a vegetarian and ate excessive amounts of fruits and vegetables. I would go years – sometimes decades – without the flu. I was the epitome of health.

But more importantly (to me) than health, I had energy.

Around the house, I did the most of the domestic duties. I vacuumed several times a week. I did the dishes twice a day. I washed the cars, washed the dogs, washed the laundry and scrubbed the bathroom - regularly.

Outside of the house, I exercised, socialized and coached.

At work, I excelled, doubling my objectives and earning more than 200K per year.

Part of my energy, I knew, was genetics. My dad is extremely energetic, so it would stand to reason I would inherit some of this.

But most of it, I believed, was will.

I *willed* myself to exercise every day. To wash the cars. To work hard. I didn't *want* to do all these things. But they needed to be done, and where there is a will, there is a way. So I *willed* myself to do those things.

Or so I believed...

BREATHLESSNESS

The first sign something might be wrong was the breathlessness.

Suddenly, I was winded when I exercised.

Not much, just a little. At first, only on the hills during family bike rides. But over time I became winded on my morning runs or when I walked the hills around the neighborhood.

This was odd. I *never* got winded. Ever.

I increased my workouts. But without effect. No matter what I did, the windedness increased, slowly but steadily. Within a couple of years, I was miserable when I did anything more than a brisk walk.

I must be getting old, I thought.   *Getting old is hell on the lungs.*

FATIGUE

Next came the fatigue.

Suddenly, I was *tired* all the time.

I went from not needing much sleep to sleeping all the time - yet never feeling rested. I'd spend all day Sunday resting in my pajamas, only to feel *more* tired on Monday.

I started letting the dishes sit, stopped washing the cars and skipped vacuuming. I felt worn down at work. I flipped out one Saturday, when my wife had the audacity to ask me to move a heavy TV ("can't I have one day to relax?" I hollered).

At first, I blamed a month-long health scare we went through with my mom. Then job stress. Then a house move. *Of course, I'm tired*, I thought. But even though the various stressful events passed, the fatigue didn't.

It kept getting worse.

BACK PAIN

As a young adult, I was prone to back pain. I would wrench my back, heal, and then wrench my back again.

Finally, when I was 24, I sprained my back lifting weights. It took a year for the sprain to completely heal, but when it did, my back troubles miraculously went away.

My back was good for the better part of 20 years.

But shortly after the fatigue set in, the back pain returned. This wasn't a wrenched back or a sprain, but a relentless lower back pain that made it difficult to even rise out of a chair.

I was doing a lot of sit ups and had changed desk chairs, so thought maybe I had pinched a nerve. I rested my back, returned to my old chair and tried back-strengthening exercises, but nothing worked.

DELUGE

For three years the symptoms – the breathlessness, the fatigue and the back pain – gradually increased. Then the dam burst.

A myriad of other symptoms came crashing down in just a few weeks of time…

I lost weight (despite eating a significant number of calories). I had stabbing chest pains and migraines every day. I developed a nagging cough that was sometimes dry and sometimes wet and speckled with blood. I was sweating through the sheets every night. And I was experiencing numbness in my arms and legs.

This wasn't aging. This wasn't stress. And this wasn't a pinched nerve.

It was time to see the doctor.

THE TESTS

In general, doctors listen. Then the better ones schedule tests (others simply dismiss the symptoms).

My GP is a good doctor. He listened. He asked questions. He did a thorough physical examination. Then he scheduled an EKG, X-ray and stress test, and before I left that first day he also drew some blood. "I don't see anything immediately scary," he said. "But let's do the tests and reconvene."

That was late Friday.

At 8:12 Monday morning, my cell phone rang. From the moment I recognized my doctor's phone number, I knew the news couldn't be good.

I answered with shaking hands.

It was my GP's assistant. "How far are you from the hospital?" she asked.

The blood test showed evidence of a pulmonary embolism. Thus began a grueling month of tests, including several hospital stays. There wasn't a pulmonary embolism but lung tests were abnormal and a high-resolution CT Scan showed "ground glass" throughout my lungs. Was it cancer? Lung disease? "It could be anything," my pulmonologist said. A lung biopsy was scheduled.

Ultimately, the lung biopsy provided a confirmed diagnosis.

I had interstitial lung disease...

THE INITIAL DIAGNOSIS

I was in and out of the hospital for a week as I recovered from my lung biopsy, which wasn't wonderful but wasn't the worst surgery I've ever had. Near the end of my stay, my surgeon checked in on me. "The lab results came back," he said. "You have Lymphoid Interstitial Pneumonia. When you are recovered we'll treat you with steroids."

"So it's curable?" I asked.

"It's treatable," he said. I smiled, happy at the news. I would not realize for several months there is a difference between *treatable* and *curable*.

LIP, as it is called, is an Interstitial Lung Disease. Interstitial means "between," and interstitial lung disease affects the tissue *between* the lung sacs instead of the actual sacs themselves. At some point my immune system convinced itself my lungs were under attack, so pumped lymphocytes into that area to isolate any toxins. Unfortunately, the lymphocytes also hamper the lung's ability to transfer oxygen into the bloodstream.

If the patient is lucky, the LIP is stabilized, meaning it doesn't get worse and - with enormous luck - may even show *some* improvement. For about half the patients, treatment doesn't work, leading to respiratory failure and other complications, usually death.

Despite the diagnosis, I wasn't worried. Most people who have LIP also have AIDS or an autoimmune disease, meaning they had underlying health issues. I'd been remarkably healthy, so I didn't think the 50% mortality rate applied to me and I fully expected to recover. I couldn't wait to start treatment.

THE "CURE"

LIP is treated with a high dosage of prednisone.

In my case this meant 50mg per day for six months, including the taper (prednisone can't simply be stopped – it has to be tapered, from 50mg to 40mg to 30mg and so on over a period of months). Anything over 20mg is considered a high dose. As I left the doctor's office with my prescription, the nurse told me, "It's unpredictable how you'll feel about the drug. Some people like the extra energy, and some people hate it." I didn't care – I just wanted treatment. But the pharmacist was a little more concerned. "Prednisone can make people paranoid," she said. "And you are on a high dose."

In my case, Prednisone was hell.

It basically shuts down the immune system – including adrenal glands – so the body can calm itself down enough to allow healing. What this meant was my body had an unnatural dose of chemicals pumping through it with no natural way for my system to control its energy levels.

Every single day for months I felt like I was trying to mask a string of all-nighters with pots of coffee – I was exhausted, foggy-headed, intensely wired and prone to instantaneous mood swings - all at the same time. Clear thought was nearly impossible, as was sleep. My hands shook, I had a puffy face (known as "moon face") and developed a rash.

But if it was hell for me, it was even more hell for my family. My mood was unpredictable. One minute I would have a flash tantrum about anything ("who left the fridge door open?!?!?!?"), then the next I was total fine, my anger completely gone ("why is everyone so upset?").

I tried everything to relax - yoga, classical music, mint tea, even listening to new age music. Nothing really helped. I just had to wait it out...

EXCITEMENT, THEN DESPAIR

May 12th, 2012 started out as a wonderful day.

The sun was shining, summer was approaching and I had completed my prednisone treatment the week before. On that day was scheduled what I thought would be my final doctor's appointment. My lungs would never be the same, but had shown remarkable levels of recovery. In my mind, LIP was a temporary scare that was ending and I could soon start the rest of my life, even though it meant my sports-playing days were over.

In many ways, I felt like I had won the lottery.

That is, I had lived.

Turns out it was just the ending of one stage – the second step in my journey was about to begin.

My doctor informed me that for at least several years, I would need regular testing. "There is just too much uncertainty," he said. In other words, there was a good chance of relapse.

I was devastated. I thought I was cured. "I don't know how you missed that," my wife told me. "I just assumed you'd have to keep going in for tests. It's like you if you had cancer."

Worse, in the weeks that followed that date, I was exhausted. I literally slept hours at a time during the day, slept 8-9 hours a night and woke up feeling more tired than I had been before I went to sleep. There would be many days where without warning I would have the uncontrollable urge to sleep. Sometimes, I'd pull the car off to the side of the road, climb into the back seat and fall almost instantly into a deep sleep for an hour or more.

This went on for weeks, then months.

Then the pain set in. Almost without warning, it felt like I had knives stabbing my knees, shoulders, back and neck. I gulped Ibuprofen four at a time, but with minimal effect.

Then my right arm stopped working. One morning, I literally couldn't lift it anymore and had to shave left handed. This was in some ways a relief -- although I couldn't feel or move my arm, at least the *pain* was gone.

I went to the doctor, who referred me to a specialist. I was diagnosed with bone spurs and pinched nerve, but the surgeon elected to wait versus proscribing surgery. "There's no guarantee the surgery will work, so I'd like to wait and see if some of the movement comes back on its own before we operate," he said. To this day I'm still grateful he waited – I'm not sure surgery would have made a difference.

Some strength gradually returned to my arm, but I still struggled to lift it above my head. But it was enough to postpone surgery indefinitely.

About the same time, my windedness started to return and my vision blurred (I went to the eye doctor, who diagnosed it as conjunctivitis, a bubbling of the eye lens).

On top of all of this, my life was in turmoil and I was suffering - mentally. I wasn't earning my bonuses anymore and the medical bills were draining away our savings. And I just didn't have the energy and focus anymore, try as though I might. I tried everything – drinking more coffee, drinking less coffee, taking more breaks, taking less breaks, changing jobs and even eating meat for the first time in four years in the hopes it might have *something* to get me going again.

Nothing helped.

Worst of all was a deep depression that settled in. "How did this all happen?" I was asking myself. "How did my life fall apart? How do I get it going again?" But the depression didn't seem *caused* by the changes – it seemed to *coincide* with them. It was something deep down inside me that I had never experienced – or imagined – before. I seemed almost physically incapable of feeling excitement or happiness, which is completely unlike me. I referred to it as, "Happiness impotent."

My doctor was perplexed. "I don't know what to tell you. Your tests are all clear."

Finally, he referred me to two specialists: a rheumatologist and a therapist.

This truly began the new chapter in my life...

"ANKLE LOOSING SPONDE – WHAT?"

My lung disease (LIP) was originally thought to be idiopathic, meaning it had no cause. It was the rheumatologist who explained that almost always LIP is caused by an autoimmune disease. LIP was not *the* condition – it was the symptom of *another* condition.

In my case, the other condition was Ankylosing Spondylitis...

I had no clue what that even was. My first thought was, *I don't have that.*

PART 2: ANKYLOSING SPONDYLITIS

AUTOIMMUNE DISEASE

Ankylosing Spondylitis is an autoimmune disease.

An autoimmune disease is essentially a whacked-out immune system. It is like the gardener who in the midst of pulling weeds starts wildly whirling his shovel, striking weeds, vegetables, fences, people – anything and everything.

A normal immune system is like an ordinary gardener -- it pulls weeds from the body. An autoimmune disease turns that gardener into a *madman* -- instead of attacking only what it's supposed to attack, it attacks itself. Skins, joints, organs – depending on the type of disease(s) – are attacked, leading to inflammation, fatigue and – often – greater complications.

One of the issues with autoimmune disease is the sufferers can appear "normal" while undergoing a private hell. Some things, like crushing fatigue, are very real consequences of autoimmune disease, but because fatigue can't be measured, it is often dismissed as being in the person's head.

There are more than 100 identified autoimmune diseases, often with similar symptoms, and these are generally treated by a rheumatologist.

Generally, autoimmune diseases are treatable but not curable. There are medicines to help slow the progression and to help with the symptoms, but the disease never goes away. Sometimes, it progresses at a steady pace regardless of treatment.

AS

In Ankylosing Spondylitis, the body attacks the spine and joints, including hips, shoulders and knees. In severe cases, AS can attack other organs, such as the intestines, eyes, heart, skin and other organs. In my case, the LIP was a matter of AS attacking my lungs. Adding to the fun, many sufferers of AS also have other autoimmune diseases, as well.

In simple terms, AS is the body figuratively kicking its own ass.

Like most autoimmune diseases, AS is incurable. Although it can go into remission and there are medicines to slow it down and treat some of the symptoms, it can't be eradicated from the system. It is always lurking.

SYMPTOMS

"Lucky" AS sufferers have very minor symptoms, primarily some back or hip pain. But many have multiple, even profound, symptoms.

On the wonderful site, Spondylitis.org, AS sufferers are invited to list their symptoms. In examining 20 postings, here were – in order – the 10 most common symptoms listed:

- Fatigue (90%)
- Hip pain (80%)
- Back pain (80%)
- Shoulder pain (80%)
- Foot and/or heel pain (80%)
- Insomnia (50%)
- Hand and/or wrist pain (50%)
- Knee pain (45%)
- Stiffness (40%)

Headaches, irritable bowels, elbow pain, leg pain, skin problems, rib pain, ankle pain, brain fog, dizziness and pain in buttocks were listed by more than 1 in 4 suffers.

In the 20 postings, 55 separate symptoms were listed at least once.

LIVING WITH AS

Living with AS can be miserable. Both physically and psychologically...

Think of those days that you are, "fighting something." On those days, you are tired. Foggy headed. Irritable. Sometimes you feel sore. The wiser people cancel their obligations, drink lots of fluids and go to bed early, hoping they feel better in the morning.

That describes a typical day when you have AS. Except for the hope. You have no chance of waking up the next day feeling "better." There is no chance of beating it.

Every single day of AS is "fighting something." And those are the good days. Because an autoimmune disease is your body perpetually "fighting something" (in this case, itself), when you have AS you generally feel crummy, tired and overwhelmed – all the time.

Sufferers are generally exhausted. They hurt. They're stiff. The pain isn't a dull ache, but often a sharp, persistent pain that varies in intensity. They suffer from "brain fog," a very real physiological response that makes clear thought almost impossible many days. Any household chore seems overwhelming and even just a coffee date can drain enough energy it takes days to recover.

I like to tell my wife that the thought of doing the dishes now is what it used to feel like when it was time to paint the house – overwhelming. Consequently, where are cars were once vacuumed – they are dirty. Piles of laundry – once unthinkable in our home – lay in our bedroom. Dirty dishes sit overnight. Sometimes I make social engagements, usually I don't. Whereas once sitting still made me literally sick to my stomach, now I spend hours at a time on the couch.

Most striking are two things: first, rest does not help me feel better, but without it, I feel worse; by worse, I mean can't think and sleep for the better part of days. Second, there is no extra gear or wells of adrenaline to reach into – when I am exhausted, I am exhausted, and there is absolutely no way to "suck it up" and "just do it." I never believed that could be true, but it is. Believe me.

For the especially lucky, the bones fuse together and the body decimates the internal organs. These folks sometimes are stooped, and often live with the specter of death (sometimes caused by a spontaneous broken spine) lingering nearby.

AS sufferers are often depressed. This actually isn't from the circumstances they live in, but an actual physiological (not psychological) symptom.

THE MENTAL DRAIN

About the same time I came down with AS, one friend broke his back and another was diagnosed with cancer. The response to both of these friends was heartwarmingly enormous – family flew in for months at a time to take care of the children, friends developed schedules for helping out around the house, neighbors developed a rotation for meals and even posted daily updates.

Although I've had some support, I've been asked many times if it's depression. People ask if I'm feeling better yet. They've said, "Maybe you're just getting older."

Such is the life when you live with a misunderstood disease. Which adds to the despair of its sufferers.

But worse is the sudden inability to do the things we all take for granted. For hanging out with friends, doing housework, even working in general. Because the person is perpetually "fighting something," and because they are hit two ways – first, their immune system is working all the time, and second their organs have to defend themselves against the attack – it is like fighting off a cold at an exponential value.

As someone who has been both exceptionally energetic and inflicted by AS, I can tell you it's impossible to imagine the depths of the fatigue. I imagine (but don't know for sure) it is a little bit like combat - you can't truly understand it unless you've experienced it.

FAMILY IMPACT

My wife has been heroic. But is has been *really* hard for her.

She is essentially married to a different man. Whereas even just a couple of short years ago I was highly energetic, highly enthusiastic, ambitious and could run the entire household by myself in addition to working full time, suddenly it's all I can do to go to work and make my way to the couch during my time off. Whereas once my relentless energy wore her down at times, now she yearns for what she had. The Monkey's Paw strikes again.

Additionally, we've seen our savings drained and our income has plummet. Every single day we see one or more medical bills, despite decent health insurance.

For friends, it has been hard to understand. They don't "get" the disease, and, to them, I *look* healthy. So they are left to wonder why I can't find the energy to hang out with them anymore. To play softball.

They can't shake the feeling that it's something psychological.

While this is hard for me, it's also hard for them. In a sense, they've lost a friend...

PART 3: FROM THE DEPTHS

For many months, I suffered. As the effects from my lung disease wore off and the fatigue dug in, I found myself sinking into the depths of depression.

Whereas I cried maybe once or twice in 20 years, I suddenly was crying every morning. "What is wrong with me," I'd ask. The pain wasn't fun, but it was the fatigue and the confusion that dragged me down.

Somehow, I was able to put on a good front, but inside I was a mess.

I was at my GP's office when he mentioned that people who had been through less than I had were farther "down" than I was. "You seem pretty buoyant," he said.

For some reason, that was a trigger. I sank. I burst into tears.

He listened, then he did two things. He put me on an antidepressant. And he referred me to a therapist.

The antidepressant helped. It wasn't the cure, but it lifted me *just enough* that the world didn't seem quite so dark. So hopeless.

Several times since then I've tried to wean myself off, but I can't. So I have given up trying – taking the medicine is just part of the after-effects of the disease.

But it was the therapist who truly lifted me out of the despair.

He listened. He validated. Then he had me focus on the positive. "Every time you start to sink," he said, "think of three things you are grateful for."

It took a while to become a habit, but now it seems natural to do.

No matter what, I can always come up with three things.

For example...

I'm alive. Several friends who were healthy when I was diagnosed haven't been so lucky. One died of an infection, another from suspected meningitis. I might not be healthy, but I'm alive. I can see my family, watch good movies and take a breath of fresh air. That's worth something.

Second, I am not on oxygen. Every 6-12 weeks I have to visit my pulmonologist. And that is a trip to reality. Every time I go, I inevitably see people of all ages in wheel chairs or carting around oxygen tanks. That could have been me, so I feel pretty lucky that it isn't.

Third, I am not hungry. Recently, I was reading about how difficult life was in the middle ages. How people were prone to disease, were under the constant threat of violent death, and lived year-to-year with the very real threat of starvation. For me, no matter how broke we might think we are, food is just a trip to the grocery store. And we always have money for food.

All over the world, there are people who'd change places with me in a heartbeat.

So I feel pretty darn lucky.

From the depths of despair, I've come to accept my life. I've come to understand that what I have is better than some, and that although I am sick, it could be a lot worse and I have a lot to be grateful for. When I think back to my early days of the disease, I realize I've come a long way mentally. And I have my therapist to thank for that.

I preach often - to *anyone* who has suffered trauma - about therapy. For anyone suffering, I think trying to find things – anything – to be grateful for is important. And, if it's at all possible, therapy is essential in overcoming the despair.

As one my doctors said, "Trying to ignore the sadness without having therapy is like trying to treat your disease by yourself."

PROLOGUE: A BETTER PERSON

SOAP BOX

If life is a journey, if it's about the experiences, than in some ways I'm grateful for my disease.

Why?

It has made me grateful.

And tolerant.

Even in my best of days, I was stressed. When I made a lot of money, I worried that I would lose the money. When I was in great shape, I worried about gaining weight. When the family was doing well, I worried about tragedy striking.

But the disease puts things in perspective. Life happens. You can't worry. We have only a few very brief cosmic moments in this world, followed by an eternity of whatever after our moments here have passed, so I'm enjoying these miracle moments while they are here. Even if I suffer from a chronic disease.

Second, it has made me more empathetic. More tolerant.

Suddenly, I understand my grandma. The crankiness, the creakiness and the despair – who am I to judge? I realize now that she probably had undiagnosed AS. The real victim was she, the person who was left to raise four children with an absent husband while likely suffering from a chronic (undiagnosed) disease. The fact she made it through that at all is heroic.

Beyond my grandma, I have more compassion for other people. I used to believe where there was a will, there was a way. Not anymore. Even "free will" is pre-disposed. Whereas I once had absolute intolerance for laziness, I now understand. Some people just weren't blessed with energy. And they may be suffering from things real or imagined that we'll never see.

Energy is a blessing – it took losing it for me to realize it.

I am grateful for so many things, mostly just to be alive. To see my kids every day, to watch a great movie, even to taste chocolate. Those are good things and I'm blessed to be here for them. Life is a good thing.

So although the disease has been hell, it has had its blessings as well. And it could be a whole lot worse. And for those times I might think otherwise, I'll make a trip to the pulmonologist. Or to the funeral home. I doubt that anyone carting around an oxygen tank or laying in a casket would give *anything* to be in my situation...

ADDED BONUSES

My disease has motivated my middle-aged wife to return to medical school. After our experience, she wants to help people who are going through what we are going through. And one thing about my wife, once she puts her mind to something, she is determined enough – and smart enough – to do it.

Additionally, my wife's going to medical school has motivated my teen daughter to become a doctor. Her grades have skyrocketed to straight As and she talks all the time about medical school.

So my experience has altered my wife and daughter's aspirations. And this may in turn help them to treat someone's illness a decade from now, who in turn may help someone else down the line.

In other words, it's impossible to know what positive impacts my illness might have in ways I can't possibly imagine.

I'm not a religious person, but I do believe in a greater purpose. And if we believe in a greater good, we have to have faith that in some way what we are going through has meaning. And we might never know what that meaning is.

We just have to have faith.

And to think of three things we are grateful for.

THE WORLD KEEPS ON TURNING

Finally, I've learned the world keeps on turning. Domestic chores might sit, work might suffer, I might have to skip socal events – but the world keeps turning.

No matter what happens and no matter what I do or don't do, the world survives and moves on.

In a strange way, this is comforting and reassuring. That is, I can be who I am right now without worrying.

COMMENTS AND RESOURCES

Please send me your thoughts! I'm at kipejennings@yahoo.com. Please remember that I suffer from fatigue, so it may take me time to respond. But I will read your note, and will respond when I can.

Also, if you send me your email (which I will not ever SPAM in any way) I will alert you when the next version is available.

I cannot recommend enough the site spondylitis.org for anyone touched by AS. It is an educational site with a tremendous number of helpful users who contribute to the forums.

50% of the proceeds from this book will go to help a student at my son's school who wants to attend a charity event in New Orleans but whose mom's health problems restricts his ability to pay for the trip (of course, this sounds nicer than it really is - for anyone not named John Grisham or Stephen King who has published a book, you know that writing a book earns maybe enough to cover the cost of a couple of martinis ☺ - but I'll funnel what comes through to him).

Thank you for your time and trust. I wish you all the best. Truly.

ABOUT THE AUTHOR

Kip Jennings is the user name of a guy who writes for the simple fun of it.

His other books – published under another pseudonym - include *My Friend Bergler, Sunriver Activities, The 10-Minute Pompeii* and *The 10-Minute Ballard.* He writes for the fun of it.

You may reach him at kipejennings@yahoo.com.

7751880R10023

Made in the USA
San Bernardino, CA
16 January 2014